SEXUALLY TRANSMITTED
INFECTIONS

The Essential Guide

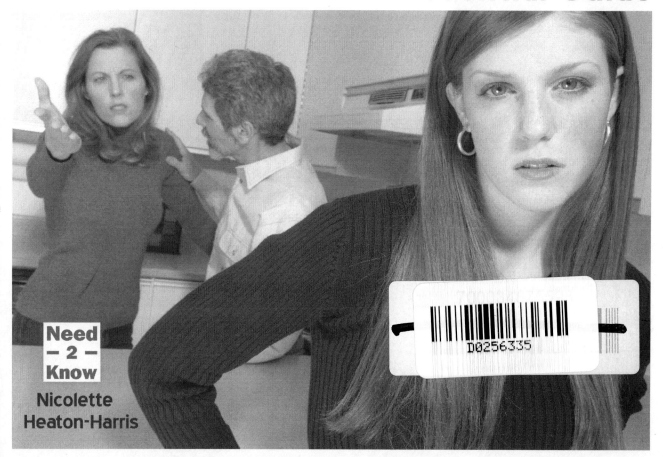

Need
– 2 –
Know

Nicolette
Heaton-Harris

D0256335

First published in Great Britain in 2008 by
Need2Know
Remus House
Coltsfoot Drive
Peterborough
PE2 9JX
Telephone 01733 898103
Fax 01733 313524
www.need2knowbooks.co.uk

Need2Know is an imprint of Forward Press Ltd.
www.forwardpress.co.uk

Contents

Acknowledgements

I would like to thank all those who gave me permission to use their information in this book, including (but not limited to) the Health Protection Agency, www.avert.org and www.embarrassingproblems.com.

I would also like to thank my family for their endless patience as I pored over medical texts, checking my facts. Any errors are my own and this book is a collection of research. I am not medically trained and I fully advise anyone who has any health concerns, sexual or otherwise, to consult with their GP.

Introduction

Sexually transmitted infections are rife in the world today. You need to arm yourself, your child, your pupil or anyone else through this sometimes deadly minefield. With this in mind, this book has been written so that you have the knowledge of the risks and the things you can do to protect yourself.

This book will guide you through the various diseases that a person, male or female, can catch from sexual contact, either vaginal, oral or anal. Let's not be coy about these matters, people do have sex in these ways and these diseases exist. Married couples, single people, young and old, male or female, any of us are at risk, and most of these infections can be disposed of easily with a course of antibiotics. Others not so easily.

Indeed there are some sexually transmitted infections (STIs) that you cannot get rid of and they can cause further health problems.

It would be quite easy to stick our heads in the sand and pretend these diseases don't exist. We could even pretend that only prostitutes or perhaps those working in the sex industry are the only people to catch these STIs – but they're not. Anyone who is sexually active is at risk of catching a sexual disease if they do not take precautions. Anyone who is casual with their health sexually, is a possible candidate for the genitourinary (GU) clinic.

This book will:

■ Guide you through the minefield of prolific infections.

■ Let you know if you're at risk of catching them.

■ Explain what you can do to prevent infection.

■ Explain about each of the infections.

■ Tell you what the signs and symptoms are.

■ Tell you what the consequences are.

■ Explain what the treatment is.

■ Explain what happens at a genitourinary (GU) clinic.

This *Essential Guide* is the definitive work on sexually transmitted infections for anyone who is sexually active and wishes to know what to do to protect themselves.

Whether you want to protect yourself, learn more about a condition you already have, or just want to know how these things are dealt with, then this is the book for you.

By the time you have read this book, you will have armed yourself with the knowledge of how to protect your sexual health and your future.

Chapter One

Chlamydia

Chlamydia (Cla – mid – ee – a) is unfortunately an extremely common sexually transmitted infection. It's a disease that has a rapidly rising detection rate in the global population, but especially in younger people.

What causes it?

Chlamydia is caused by a bacterium, known as chlamydia trachomatis. This particular strain of the bacteria can cause non-specific urethritis (inflammation of the urethra) in men, pelvic inflammatory disease (PID) in women and inclusion conjunctivitis in a newborn baby (symptoms are apparent five to 13 days after the birth).

Chlamydia can seriously damage a woman's reproductive organs before any symptoms are ever noticed. It is often referred to as a 'silent' disease, because many women do not even know they have it until they go to a hospital or doctor to be treated for something else. Future fertility can be seriously compromised by this disease, so if any symptoms are noticed, it is imperative that you receive treatment.

In a man, chlamydia can cause a discharge from the penis, so men would have to be aware for any penile changes.

Is chlamydia that common?

Chlamydia is the most commonly detected and reported sexually transmitted infection in the United Kingdom today. It is believed that 1 in 10 females under the age of 25 is possibly infected and most of them do not know they have the condition. Unfortunately, this also means that the rate of chlamydia infection could be a lot higher, as most people who have chlamydia don't even know

'Chlamydia is one of the most prevalent sexually transmitted infections in our society today.'

they have it, so it leads to less cases being reported than there actually are. The Centre for Disease Control (CDC) estimate that in America, 2.8 million people (male and female) are infected with chlamydia each year and a lot of females get re-infected because their partners are not treated.

Whichever sexually transmitted infection a person gets, they must always inform their current and past sexual partners and insist that they get tested and, if required, treated.

'Chlamydia is often known as the "silent disease" as there are often no symptoms. Many women do not know they have it until they go to a hospital or doctor to be treated for something else.'

How am I going to catch it?

You can be infected by chlamydia through vaginal, oral or anal sex. Chlamydia trachoma can also be transmitted from a mother to a newborn baby as it passes through the birth canal, causing an eye irritation (inclusion conjunctivitis).

The least you need to know is that if you are sexually active in any way at all, then you are at risk of being infected by chlamydia if the person you are with is knowingly or unknowingly infected. If you have more than one sexual partner, then your risk is naturally higher.

If you are male and have either oral or anal sex with a male or female, then you are also at risk of infection as this disease can be passed through oral and anal sex too.

Younger women and girls are particularly vulnerable it seems because their cervix (the opening to the uterus) has not fully matured and is more vulnerable to infection by the chlamydial bacteria. If you have a teenage daughter who you know is sexually active, then it is important that you inform her of this fact. Tips on how to talk to your teenager are included at the end of this chapter.

What symptoms should I be looking out for?

If you have chlamydia, you may not always know about it. This disease is called a 'silent' disease because it is thought that about 75% of those infected have no symptoms whatsoever. However, if you do experience the symptoms that follow, you will tend to notice them appearing about one to three weeks after your initial infection, so it is imperative that you think back to which partner or partners you were with.

Need2Know

Symptoms in women:

- An abnormal vaginal discharge.
- A burning sensation when urinating.
- Lower abdominal pain.
- Lower back pain.
- Nausea.
- Raised temperature / fever.
- Pain during sex.
- Bleeding between periods.

While these symptoms are being experienced, the infection is usually spreading from the cervix, where it tends to originate, to the fallopian tubes (the tubes that carry eggs from the ovaries to the womb).

Symptoms in men:

- Abnormal discharge from the penis.
- A burning sensation when urinating.
- A burning feeling around the opening of the penis.
- Itching around the opening of the penis.

Rarely do men experience pain and swelling in their testicles with chlamydial infection.

If you have anal sex and are infected with chlamydia, you can experience from the rectum:

- Rectal pain.
- Abnormal discharge.
- Bleeding.

Of course any bleeding or strange discharge from the rectum should always be investigated anyway to remove any possibilities of a more serious bowel problem.

Those of you who indulge in oral sex with a partner infected with chlamydia, can expect to experience a very sore and painful throat.

So what will happen if I don't get this treated?

Unfortunately, if chlamydia goes undiagnosed for a very long time, then serious problems affecting future fertility and health can present themselves.

A woman may discover that she has developed pelvic inflammatory disease (PID). PID can be either an acute (short term) or chronic (long term) condition. If you have PID, then your uterus, fallopian tubes and ovaries are going to be infected; they become inflamed by the presence of infection from another place (usually the site of infection – the cervix).

PID is usually suspected after a woman experiences lower abdominal pain that can sometimes be quite severe.

Acute (short term) infections can often be treated with antibiotics, but if you are affected by a chronic (long term) condition of PID, then pelvic adhesions (the joining of two usually separate organs) can form and surgical intervention is then necessary to remove any affected tissue. Very often the fallopian tubes can become blocked, leading to an ectopic pregnancy and lowered fertility. Alarmingly, the Centre for Disease Control (CDC) estimates that up to 40% of women with untreated chlamydia will develop PID.

If you are a woman and are infected with chlamydia, then you are also at greater risk of contracting HIV, if exposed to it.

If you are a man, then complications from chlamydial infection are less common (or reported). Sometimes the infection can spread to the epididymis (a seven metre long tube that connects the testes to the vas deferens. The epididymis provides the route through which sperm matures over a period of days before ejaculation). This causes a condition called epididymitis, in which the infection has spread down the vas deferens from the urethra, resulting in pain, swelling and a redness of the affected area. You may experience a fever and in some rare cases, sterility. Sometimes this infection may spread down to the testicle, but it can be treated by antibiotics.

'Chlamydia can be responsible for non-specific urethritis in men, pelvic inflammatory disease (PID) in women and inclusion conjunctivitis in the newborn.'
Oxford Medical Dictionary, OUP, 2003.

Occasionally, chlamydial infection can cause arthritis and skin lesions such as Reiter's Syndrome (named after the German doctor who discovered it.) Reiter's Syndrome is an inflammation of the urethra, conjunctivitis, and polyarthritis that usually, but not always, affects young men. The aim of treating Reiter's is to reduce the pain caused by the inflammation. Non-steroidal anti-inflammatories (NSAIDs) are mainly used.

I'm pregnant. How does having chlamydia affect me?

Chlamydia will not affect the baby until it passes through the birth canal; however, there is some evidence that points to some women experiencing premature delivery while being affected by chlamydia. When the baby passes through the birth canal, the bacteria from the infection affects the baby's eyes and respiratory tracts and has been reported as a leading cause of early infant pneumonia and pink eye.

How will a doctor test me for chlamydia?

When you go to see your doctor (or go to the GU clinic), there are two ways they can test for chlamydia infection. You can provide them with a urine sample which they will send to their laboratory for testing, or they will painlessly take a swab from your penis or cervix and send that off for testing instead.

If my result is positive, what treatment will I have?

Chlamydia, caught early, is easily treated and, more importantly, it's cured with a simple course of antibiotics. The two most common drugs used are Azithromycin and Doxycycline. Azithromycin (trade name – Zithromax) is taken by mouth in a single dose. The possible side effects include nausea and allergic reaction.

Doxycycline (trade name – Vibramycin) is also administered orally, twice daily, usually over seven days. It is a tetracycline and its possible side effects include sickness or diarrhoea.

If you are HIV positive, then you will be treated the same as if you were HIV negative.

Once your diagnosis of chlamydia has been made, it is crucial that all of your sexual partners are notified, tested and treated. A positive result means that you should abstain from sexual intercourse until you and your partner / partners have completed all your antibiotics, otherwise re-infection with the disease is more than likely.

Re-infection is not something that should be taken lightly, especially in a woman. Multiple infections with chlamydia increase a woman's risk of infertility and future complications. Women should strongly consider getting themselves re-tested for chlamydia 12 to 16 weeks after completing a treatment. Not only will this put your mind at rest, but it will also let you know if your partner has received treatment.

How can I protect myself against chlamydia?

Abstaining from sex is the easiest way, but sometimes this is not appropriate. Many of you may be married or in a long-term relationship. Sex can play a huge part in many relationships and it is important to a lot of people, even if they're not strictly 'committed'.

If you are in a monogamous relationship, make sure that your partner has been tested and that they are uninfected. If you are male, ensure you wear a condom – if used correctly and every time, this alone can reduce the risk of chlamydia transmission.

If you are female, sexually active and under the age of 25, then you can participate in chlamydia screening annually. This also applies to older women who have a new sexual partner or multiple partners. You can have your risk factors assessed at your doctor's surgery or at your local GU clinic. If you are pregnant, then you will – hopefully – be tested for chlamydia as a matter of course.

The main thing to remember is that if you have any change in genital symptoms – discharge, burning, itching, sores, rashes, lumps, etc – it should be a clear cut sign to you that there is a problem and you should abstain from sex until you have sorted the problem by visiting your GP or GU clinic.

How do I talk to my teenager about sex and infection?

It can be difficult for a parent to decide to talk to their teenager about sex. Some of you may want to get the conversation over and done with really quickly out of embarrassment, so it can be quite an easy mistake to stick to the basics and not mention all the extras that come with the subject.

Sexually transmitted infections may not be something you want to talk about at all. You may have a strong belief that there should be no sex before marriage. You may believe that your teenage son or daughter should not have sex unless they are deeply in love with their choice of partner. You may believe that sex is simply a pure thing; a beautiful gift and you want your child to believe it too. Therefore you're really reluctant to talk about all the diseases out there; diseases that may sully their idea of sex and love.

Unfortunately, whether you like it or not, many teenagers today have sex. They may do it to:

- Lose their virginity.
- Keep up with their friends.
- Be accepted.
- Keep a boyfriend / girlfriend.

They may get drunk at a party and it just happens.

You may not want to admit that this kind of thing happens, but it does. You prepare your child for many other things in life, so why not prepare them for sex? Why not protect them from the various diseases that are out there at the same time?

We prepare our children for school – we protect them from bullies.

We prepare our children to drive – we get them insured, give them driving lessons and help them buy a car.

Why not prepare them for sex by giving them the knowledge to do it right? To protect themselves when it happens. Forewarning them, is forearming them, isn't it?

Talking to your child about sex, about condoms, about protection, about infection, is not letting them think they can go off and have loads of sex. This is not a subject you should be shy about. Don't even believe you're the first person to talk to them about this.

Children today are exposed to sexual imagery and information from quite an early age. They see it on television and on their computers. It's in their computer games and in magazines and newspapers. Their friends will have talked to them about it. They will have laughed and joked about it. Giggled and blushed about it. But will they have been given guidance about it?

This is part of your job as a responsible parent. Only you know your child. Only you will know whether it's best to sit in your child's room to talk about this or whether to take them out somewhere and talk. The key is knowing your child well enough to decide where the best place for that talk is.

Below are a few points you need to make clear with them.

- If they choose to have sex, they must do it safely.
- Safe sex means always using a condom.
- They can become infected with chlamydia if their partner is infected, which means they could catch a disease the first time they have sex.
- They should be aware of their own bodies and be able to note any changes such as a discharge.
- Chlamydia, if left untreated, can severely affect their future sexual health and fertility.
- Chlamydia can be caught through oral and vaginal sex, as well as anal.
- They must not have sex with their partner if that partner is still under treatment for chlamydia.
- If they are unsure, then they should abstain from sex and stay safe.
- They should never allow themselves to be pressured into having sex without a condom.

Factfile

Chlamydia has one of the fastest growing rates of infection in our society today. Some experts believe that this growth in infection rates has something to do with our binge-drinking culture, as alcohol lowers inhibitions and makes people take risks that they would not normally take when sober, e.g. having sex impulsively and without using condoms.

One GU clinic in the Portsmouth area of the UK had 1,360 reported cases of chlamydia in the year 2002. But, in 2006, this figure had skyrocketed to 2,421 reported cases; an increase of 78%. (*Portsmouth News*, 2007.)

According to a report by the Health Protection Agency, there were 42,668 reported cases of uncomplicated chlamydia in 1997. This figure rose to 68,332 in 2000 and rose dramatically again in 2006 to 113,585 cases; a massive rise of 166%.

Summing Up

- Chlamydia is a bacterial infection that can be treated, if caught early enough, with a simple course of antibiotics.

- Chlamydia can be tested for by means of a simple swab or urine test.

- Chlamydia can be transmitted through vaginal, anal or oral sex.

- Chlamydia is one of the most prevalent sexually transmitted infections in our society today.

- If in doubt about your partner's sexual health, then abstain from sex.

- Always use a condom, especially with a new sexual partner.

Chapter Two

Gonorrhoea

Gonorrhoea (gon – nor – ree – a) is a sexually transmitted infection caused by a bacteria that affects the mucous membranes in the genital area of either sex. It grows easily in moist, warm areas, so the reproductive tract, cervix, womb, fallopian tubes and urethra in women give it a perfect environment in which to spread. In men, gonorrhoea tends to infect the urethra, but the bacteria can also grow in a person's mouth, throat, eyes and anus.

How common is gonorrhoea?

Gonorrhoea is unfortunately very common and you are at risk if you do not have safe sex. Symptoms do not generally appear until a week after infection, so it can easily be spread if a person has more than one sexual partner within a week of being infected. Gonorrhoea affects members of either sex.

How am I going to catch it?

The gonorrhoea bacteria are passed through sexual contact with the penis, vagina, anus or mouth. A man does not have to ejaculate for it to pass to his partner. Simple contact is all that is required. If you are pregnant and you have gonorrhoea, then you will be able to pass it to your baby during the delivery through the birth canal. Gonorrhoea can be treated with antibiotics, but once your infection has cleared up, this does not mean you will be immune from contracting gonorrhoea again.

'The Centre for Disease Control (CDC) estimates that more than 700,000 people are infected with gonorrhoea each year in America alone, yet only half of these are reported.'
Centre for Disease Control and Prevention, www.cdc.gov/std/ Gonorrhea/STDFact- gonorrhea.htm.

What symptoms should I be looking out for?

Symptoms develop about one week after the initial infection and include:

- Pain on passing urine.
- A discharge of white, yellow or green pus from the penis or vagina.
- In men, sometimes there is pain or swelling in the testicles.
- Vaginal bleeding between periods in women.

Rectal infection symptoms include:

- Anal discharge.
- Anal itching.
- Soreness.
- Bleeding.
- Painful bowel movements.

Sometimes, there may be no signs of infection at all, which is why it is very important to have sexual health screening not only for you, but for any future partner. Women can sometimes mistake a gonorrhoea infection for a bladder infection and if they do not get treated correctly, are at risk of severe complications.

Gonorrhoea infection in the throat after oral sex can cause a painful throat, but no other symptoms.

It has also been known for signs of gonorrhoeal infection to appear up to a month after the initial infection.

So what will happen if I don't get this treated?

There are many complications to consider and some of them are quite serious. In untreated cases, the infection may spread throughout the reproductive system, causing sterility in both males and females. In women, gonorrhoea can also cause pelvic inflammatory disease (PID – see the information in previous chapter).

In men, gonorrhoea can develop severe inflammation of the urethra to such an extent that it prevents the passage of urine, a condition known as stricture.

Stricture is the name given to any narrowing of a tubular structure within the body, such as the urethra. When a urethral stricture occurs, the urethra itself narrows as a result of its inflammation and the man has difficulty in passing urine and possibly develops retention (acute retention can be painful, whereas chronic retention can become painless).

The stricture must then be assessed by a doctor in a procedure called an urethrography. This is an x-ray examination of the urethra, which involves a contrast medium, usually a dye, being passed into the urethra so that its outline and narrowing / abnormalities can be seen. The contrast dye is injected into the urethra using a special syringe and a penile clamp. A doctor can also assess the stricture using a urethroscope (an endoscope, shaped like a very fine tube, fitted with a light and a lens for interior examination of the urethra).

During a urethroscopy, periodic dilation (widening) of the urethra is performed using sounds, urethrotomy (cutting a stricture in the urethra, using a fine blade passed down through the endoscope) or urethroplasty (inserting a flap or patch of skin from the scrotum or perineum into the urethra at the site of the stricture). The urethroplasty can be done in one stage, but usually a doctor may choose to do it in two stages if they are repairing a ruptured posterior urethral stricture.

'If left totally untreated, gonorrhoea can be life-threatening.'

Men are also at risk of contracting epididymitis (see previous chapter).

In both sexes, gonorrhoeal infection can also spread to the blood and joints. Later complications can include arthritis, inflammation of the heart valves (endocarditis; a temporary or permanent damage to the heart valves which can result from this infection. Symptoms include fever, heart murmurs, heart failure and embolism. Endocarditis can be treated with antibiotics, but surgery may be required to repair damaged heart valves) and infection of the eyes (conjunctivitis; red, swollen eyes with a pus/watery discharge). If left totally untreated, gonorrhoea can be life-threatening.

If you contract gonorrhoea, then you are at a higher risk of contracting HIV, the virus that causes AIDS. Those infected with HIV and gonorrhoea can more easily pass HIV on to an uninfected person than if they did not have gonorrhoea.

I'm pregnant. How does having gonorrhoea affect me?

If you are pregnant and have gonorrhoea, then you are at risk of passing the infection into the eyes of your baby as it passes down through the birth canal. This condition is known as ophthalmia neonatorum. The two most common infections to cause this condition in a baby are chlamydia and gonorrhoea. If the infection in the baby's eyes is not treated, then it can sometimes cause:

- Permanent eye disease.
- Blindness.
- Joint infection.
- Or a life-threatening blood infection in the baby.

'A pregnant woman can pass gonorrhoea onto her baby.'

It can be easily diagnosed by a quick swab of the affected area and is treated with antibiotics for both mother and baby.

How will a doctor test me for gonorrhoea?

There are different ways that a doctor or clinic can test for gonorrhoea. A swab can be taken from any part of the body thought to be infected such as the cervix, rectum, throat, vagina or urethra and then the swab will be sent away for analysis. If gonorrhoea is suspected in the area of the cervix or urethra, then a urine sample will be adequate for testing.

A doctor or clinic may choose to use a Gram Stain to test for gonorrhoea. For a Gram Stain, a film of possible bacteria is spread across a glass slide, dried and heat-fixed with a violet-coloured dye, then treated with a decolouriser (alcohol), then counter-stained with a red dye. Gram negative bacteria lose the initial stain, but take up the second so they appear red, whereas Gram positive bacteria keep the initial stain and appear violet. A Gram Stain is usually used to test men, rather than women as the test seems to work better on males.

If my result is positive, what treatment will I receive?

Gonorrhoea is treated with antibiotics. Ciprofloxacin, Ofloxacin or Cefotaxime are usually quite effective in combating the bacteria.

Ciprofloxacin (trade names – Ciloxan or Ciproxin) is a broad-spectrum quinolone antibiotic that is very useful in treating bacteria that are Gram-negative and resistant to other oral antibiotics. Possible side effects include nausea, diarrhoea, stomach pains or headache. It is also used in the treatment of eye infections.

Ofloxacin (trade names – Exocin or Tarivid) is another quinolone antibiotic specifically used to treat urinary tract and sexually transmitted infections. It can be administered orally or by injection. Possible side effects include sickness and skin rashes.

How can I protect myself against catching gonorrhoea?

The easiest way, as always, is to abstain from sex! But, as mentioned before, this isn't always an easy matter, depending upon your relationship. Always use condoms if you have more than one partner, or change partner frequently. But, if you are in a long-term monogamous relationship, using condoms is usually the safest way if you have both been tested and the results were negative.

Always use a condom when having sex and if you notice any difference in your genital area, or suspect an unusual discharge, then you must always get it investigated. Any strange symptom 'down below' should be a direct and immediate signal to stop having sex immediately until an infection has been discounted. This should help reduce risks for both yourself and your partner.

'Anyone who is sexually active can be at risk from gonorrhoea infection.'

Talking to a teenager about gonorrhoea

Usually just the mention of sex or a 'dirty infection' is enough to get them giggling, so it is imperative that you make them understand how serious an infection like gonorrhoea is.

Let them know that it isn't just prostitutes who catch this. It isn't just people that sleep around a lot who catch this. It's a risk for anyone and they need to know the signs and symptoms and how to avoid catching it.

Tell them they must:

* Always wear a condom.

* Not be promiscuous.

* Insist on safe sex with every partner.

Gonorrhoea isn't just 'the clap'. It's not just something dirty that they ought to keep quiet about or can get rid of when they get round to going to the doctors. They shouldn't be embarrassed. This isn't just about an infection. It could be their life.

Factfile

Infection rates for gonorrhoea are on the rise after an initial decline during the 1970s.

At the GU clinic in Portsmouth, they had 1,121 reported cases of gonorrhoea during 2002, but, by 2006, that figure had risen to 1,269 reported cases; an increase of 13%. (*Portsmouth News*, 2007.)

That may not seem much when you compare it to the rate of increase reported with chlamydial infections, but remember these were reported infections. How many people were too embarrassed to go to see their doctor and preferred to keep quiet?

According to a report by the Health Protection Agency, there were 13,063 cases of gonorrhoea in the UK during 1997 which rose by 46% to 19,007 reported cases in 2006.

Summing Up

- Gonorrhoea will thrive and quickly grow to infect areas such as the reproductive tract, the cervix, the womb, fallopian tubes and the urethra in men.

- It is spread through simple genital contact.

- Ejaculation is not required for gonorrhoea to spread.

- Some men with gonorrhoea may have no symptoms at all.

- In women, the symptoms of gonorrhoea can be mild and mistaken for bladder infections.

- Complications from undiagnosed and untreated gonorrhoea can cause serious health problems.

- Gonorrhoea passed to a baby can cause blindness and other serious health issues.

- Antibiotics can be used to treat gonorrhoea, but there are some antibiotic-resistant strains.

- Latex condoms can be an effective prevention against gonorrhoea, but do not provide 100% protection.

Chapter Three

Genital Herpes

Genital Herpes (gen – it – ul – her – pees) is a sexually transmitted infection caused by the herpes simplex viruses type 1 (HSV-1) and type 2 (HSV-2). Both types cause an inflammation of the skin or mucous membranes and are generally observed by displaying collections of small blisters.

HSV-1 causes the cold sore that you often see around someone's mouth, whereas HSV-2 is mainly associated with genital herpes and is sexually transmitted. However, both HSV-1 and HSV-2 can cause either cold sores or genital herpes, depending upon where and how the infection takes place.

What is genital herpes?

Genital herpes can be contracted by either of the viruses described above, but some people show no signs of having it at all, or have just a few indications that there is 'something' present.

When there are signs, the things to look for are one or more blisters on or around the genitals or anus of either sex. These blisters do break, which leave very tender and often sore ulcers that can take from a fortnight to a month to heal from the first outbreak. Usually, a secondary outbreak can appear weeks or months after the first set of blisters, but, this secondary set is often less pronounced, less severe in tenderness and the outbreak tends to last a shorter amount of time.

This infection can stay in the body, yet the outbreaks can get less and less as time passes.

How am I going to catch it?

Both HSV-1 and HSV-2 are in the sores that they create and are released from the blisters as well as from patches of skin that do not appear to be broken or have sores. This is how individuals who have no sign of infection still manage to infect others.

You can only get an HSV-2 infection during sexual contact with a person who is already infected with HSV-2.

HSV-1 can still cause genital herpes as stated previously, but it more commonly causes the sore blisters about the mouth. HSV-1 infection around the genitals can be caused by oral-genital contact with a person who has a visible or not HSV-1 infection. HSV blisters are highly contagious.

'Herpes can seem severe in people who already have a suppressed immune system.'

What symptoms should I be looking out for?

A lot of men and women infected with the HSV-2 strain are unfortunately unaware of their infection. However, if they do have an outbreak, the first one can be quite pronounced and will hopefully make them seek medical intervention and treatment.

The first outbreak of blisters usually occurs about a fortnight after the initial transmission of infection and then those sores usually heal about a fortnight to a month afterwards.

Other signs and symptoms at the first outbreak can include:

▪ A second amount of fresh sores immediately after the first is noticed.

▪ Fever.

▪ Swollen glands.

However, many people with an HSV-1 infection don't actually get any sores, or they have mild signs of a skin problem that they could mistake for a heat rash or insect bites.

If you are diagnosed with genital herpes, then you can expect to have (typically, but not always) four or five further recurrences of sores within that first year after infection. These outbreaks will then decrease over time, though the virus may remain present, yet dormant, in the body.

So what will happen if I don't get this treated?

Herpes simplex virus can also affect the conjunctiva in the eyes and form what is called a dendritic ulcer. The surface of the cornea in the eye develops an ulcer and these can continually reoccur as the virus lies in the tissues of the body between attacks.

If you have a suppressed or weakened immune system then contracting a herpes infection can be serious as your body will struggle to fight the infection. There is also a large problem psychologically for people infected with herpes and they can suffer huge amounts of distress, which should not be overlooked.

But the biggest problem by far is that genital HSV infection can cause a potentially fatal infection in a baby carried by a pregnant woman, though fortunately, this occurrence is extremely rare and if a woman is known to have genital herpes while pregnant, a doctor will advise a caesarean section.

Herpes is also suspected of assisting the spread of HIV, the virus that spreads AIDS.

'Herpes may play a role in the spread of HIV.' Centre for Disease Control and Prevention, www.cdc. gov/std.

I'm pregnant. How does having herpes affect me?

If you are pregnant, it is incredibly important that you do not contract herpes. It can cause a fatal infection in a child and having your first outbreak of sores while pregnant creates a greater risk of transmission to the baby.

If your genital herpes is active at the time of delivery, then your doctors will perform a caesarean section to help protect the baby.

How will a doctor test me for herpes?

If you suspect you may have herpes, then your doctor can visually examine you and the site of infection, if the outbreak is currently active, and then take a sample from a sore for testing in a laboratory. If your sores are not currently active, then it can be harder to diagnose but not impossible.

A sample of blood can be sent for testing both HSV-1 and HSV-2, but these are not always 100% accurate.

'The surest way to avoid transmission of genital herpes is to abstain from sex, or be in a long term monogamous relationship with someone whom you know has been tested and is free of infection.'

If my result is positive, how will I be treated?

Unfortunately there is no definitive cure for herpes simplex virus, but a doctor can prescribe you some anti-viral medications that can shorten and help try to prevent outbreaks while the medication is taken. There are also some suppressive therapies that have to be taken daily if you want to reduce the risk of transmitting herpes to a partner.

All forms of herpes are treated with Aciclovir (trade name – Zovirax) or another anti-viral drug. Aciclovir is an anti-viral drug that prevents DNA synthesis in the cells inhabited by the herpes viruses. It can be taken orally or by IV (intravenously through a vein), affecting herpes zoster (shingles), genital herpes, herpetic eye disease and herpes encephalitis (inflammation of the brain).

How can I protect myself against herpes?

The surest way is to avoid sexual contact or be in a long term monogamous relationship with someone whom you know has been tested and is free of infection. However, this is not always easy to achieve.

The ulcers around the genitals in men can be covered partially by a condom, but a condom will not always cover the areas infected and herpes can be spread from the skin that does not appear to have sores. Obviously, the correct and consistent use of latex condoms will go some way to partially protecting you against herpes, but will not guarantee full protection.

If you or your partner has an active outbreak of sores, then you should abstain from sex definitely during that period, both genitally and orally. Remember, an infected partner can still transmit the virus when the sores are not present.

You should always be aware of your own health and that of your sexual partner and if there are any suspicions at all, then abstaining from sex is the only sure way to protect you from infection. You can go to your doctor or a GU clinic and ask to be tested even if you show no signs of genital herpes. A positive blood test definitely indicates infection with HSV-2.

Talking to a teenager about genital herpes

Herpes as a subject is one that can greatly confuse some young people. They see a friend with a cold sore and sometimes assume that their friend must have had oral sex to catch it. This is not always the case and you must make sure they understand this, explaining about HSV-1 and HSV-2.

If you hear your own child talking about sex, say on their mobile phone, then wait until they come off their phone and are on their own before asking them questions about it. Don't harass them. Be genuinely interested and make sure that they know exactly what they're talking about. Some young teenagers bandy words around that other teenagers use and sometimes aren't exactly sure of their definition.

A good website for parents is www.urbandictionary.com which gives a brief and easy explanation of current uses of slang and 'in' words used by the youth of today. (See page 93 for more on this.)

If you feel that after talking to your child that they may be at risk sexually, then make sure you inform them about protection. Condoms are freely available at some clinics, but in the case of herpes, condoms will not always be 100% effective.

But can you guarantee they will abstain from sex because you don't want them to be having intercourse? Can you watch your teenager 24 hours a day?

It's mostly impossible to do this. So arm them with the knowledge they need to protect their health and futures.

Factfile

Cases of genital herpes are rising steadily, not just here in the United Kingdom, but across the globe.

In 1997, the Health Protection Agency reported that there were 16,615 cases of genital herpes (these were first attacks of the condition and do not include those people who have returned at a later date, re-infected). By the millennium (2000), there were a reported 17,823 cases. Three years later in 2003, this had risen again to 19,231 cases, and in 2006 it had increased to 21,698 reports of genital herpes; an increase of 31% from 1997.

Summing Up

- There are two types of herpes simplex virus, HSV-1 and HSV-2.

- Most infected individuals have no visible signs of infection.

- Visible signs can include blisters and sores around the genitals.

- Secondary outbreaks can appear less severe than the first.

- Genital herpes can also cause sores around the mouth.

- An infected person can expect to have four or five outbreaks in their first year.

- Herpes is generally diagnosed by taking a sample from an open sore.

- HSV-2 infection is generally more common in women.

- No treatment can currently cure herpes, but it can be treated.

- You should never have sex if you know your partner is infected.

- Because of the visible signs of herpes, this infection can cause psychological distress as well as physical upset.

Chapter Four

Genital Warts

A wart is a non-cancerous growth on the surface of the skin, ranging in size from 1-10mm in diameter and is mainly found on the hands. However, genital warts (gen – it – ul – warts) are often associated with other sexual, genital infections and in women are associated with an increased risk of cervical cancer.

What causes genital warts?

Genital warts are caused by the human papillomavirus (HPV). There are differing types of HPV and some of them simply cause the genital wart, whilst others are associated with causing certain cancers in both males and females in and around their genital area.

So what does the human papillomavirus do?

A member of the papovavirus group (DNA containing a virus capable of producing tumours in animals and humans), HPV causes warts. There are over 50 strains of the virus and certain strains are associated with causing anal and cervical cancers (though other conditions also have to be present).

Are genital warts common?

Unfortunately so; rates of incidence of this infection have risen by a third in the last few years. In one study, all the women in a college were tested for HPV and 50% returned positive tests, yet only 1-2% showed any signs of infection.

Infection with HPV is common, but yet again, not many people will actually show any signs of infection.

What symptoms should I be looking out for?

Well, obviously, warts. These do not always appear on the outside of the body on the external genitalia, but inside on the inner walls of the vagina or even higher up on or around the cervix.

What will happen if I don't get them treated?

If you choose not to get your genital warts treated, then there are some serious possible complications that might occur. Genital warts are not like the warts you get on your hands where they usually go away on their own after a couple of years.

For women, there is a higher risk of being vulnerable to cervical cancer. Regular cervical smear tests are essential in these cases, as in the presence of HPV there is a tendency towards a higher risk of a woman developing premalignant cell abnormalities. Ensuring that as a woman you have regular smear tests, these possible changes can be detected early and treated.

However, the risk of cancer from genital warts is not just confined to women. Men can also be at risk from penile cancers. There are different cells within the body of the penis and all of them can be affected by different types of cancers. The two most commonly seen are epidermoid carcinoma (affecting the skin of the penis) and verrucous carcinoma (affecting the cells themselves). There is a third, but rare cancer of the penis, adenocarcinoma (affecting the sweat glands of the penis). All penile cancers are treated in different ways, but patients can expect either radiation therapy, chemotherapy, surgery or a mixture of all three.

Cervical cancer - what should I know?

Let me reiterate that just because someone has genital warts, it does not mean that they will definitely get cervical cancer. But they do have a higher risk.

Cervical carcinoma is when a cancer develops in the neck of the uterus (the cervix). A tumour may develop, which can also become invasive, spreading to surrounding tissues and subsequently into the lymphatic system and lymph nodes. Organs close by, such as the bladder, the bowel and rectum will be at a high risk.

Cancer of the cervix can be detected really early if a woman has regular smears. Sometimes there can also be symptoms, such as a vaginal discharge that smells or is blood stained.

Treatment for this cancer can be by irradiation (radiotherapy), surgery or both. Certain cytotoxic drugs (drugs used to treat cancers) may also be used.

I'm pregnant. How does having warts affect me?

If your baby passes through the birth canal while you have warts, then it is possible that the baby may become infected.

How will a doctor test me for warts?

You can see your own doctor or go to a clinic if you suspect genital warts. However, if you have no visible symptoms, but suspect you are infected, then there are some simple ways you can get diagnosed.

A visual examination by a doctor can confirm the presence of warts, but if you have no visible signs then some more invasive procedures may be required.

A doctor may perform a colposcopy. This involves a doctor inserting a colposcope into the vagina, permitting a more thorough visual examination of the cervix and upper part of the vagina.

There is also a DNA test that can be used, that is highly effective in detecting HPV in an apparently infection-free person. This test, called a polymerase chain reaction (PCR) can give very accurate results. PCR examines a particular sequence of DNA in the genes, amplifying it to detect viruses in human tissue samples, such as HPV in cervical smears.

I've tested positive for warts. What treatment will I have?

Treatment for warts can be relatively simple for the visible warts around the genitals. Over the counter products can be used; especially those that contain lactic and salicylic acids (a drug that causes the human skin to peel off. It kills bacteria and fungi beneath the skin. However, if you have very sensitive skin, then there can be a reaction if you have to continually reapply the treatment). However, freezing the warts using cryotherapy with liquid nitrogen is probably going to be the most effective and responsive treatment.

Sometimes, a doctor may suggest curettage (using a spoon-shaped instrument to scrape the skin) and cautery (killing tissue using heat).

How can I protect myself against warts?

If you are sexually active, then you cannot guarantee yourself 100% protection from warts, especially if you have been with a new partner or multiple partners. The best way is to abstain from sex.

You are at increased risk of genital warts if you have:

- Multiple partners.
- Have sex at an early age.
- If you smoke.
- If you are malnourished.
- If you suffer from stress.
- If you have other genital infections.
- If you have a viral infection.
- If you have HIV.

If your partner does not visibly have any signs of genital warts, then this cannot guarantee that they are not infected with HPV. Only if you have both been tested and you are in a monogamous long term relationship are you considered relatively safe from contracting genital warts. Condoms will not be able to give you 100% protection from this infection.

Talking to a teenager about genital warts

One thing to make clear when talking to a teenager about the various infections is that they know the differences.

Many teenagers will believe that genital warts and genital herpes are exactly the same thing, but with just a different name for some reason! Make it clear that these are two completely different viruses. Herpes may be unpleasant and embarrassing, but genital warts can cause, with a combination of other risk factors, cancer. Your teenager must understand the huge implications of these ugly little bumps that may or may not be there.

Factfile

In the Portsmouth area alone, the rate of cases of genital warts has increased by 35% in just four years. (*Portsmouth News*, 2007.)

Nationwide in the UK, according to a report by the Health Protection Agency, in 1997 there were 68,883 reported cases of first infections of genital warts. This number rose to 71,317 by 2000, and in 2006 had reached an incredible 83,745 new cases; a 22% increase.

Obviously this infection is on the rise, but the possibility of a new vaccine being introduced in the future may help reduce the number of new infections.

'Herpes may be unpleasant and embarrassing, but genital warts can cause, with a combination of other risk factors, cancer.'

Summing Up

- Genital warts can be found on the genitalia of either sex, around the anus, or internally.

- As genital warts are usually spread through sexual contact, any young child with genital warts should be thoroughly investigated to rule out abuse.

- Getting rid of warts can involve either topical medications or the use of surgical techniques.

- If you are a woman and you have, or have had, warts then you should ensure that you have more regular cervical smears than a woman who is negative for genital warts.

- Genital warts can put a sufferer at a higher risk for cancer.

Chapter Five

Syphilis

(Sif – fill – lis) is a sexually transmitted infection caused by a bacterium known as treponema pallidum (this bacterium grows without the presence of oxygen and has a flexible, spiral shape). This infection is chronic, which means that it is long-lasting, rather than an acute condition which lasts for only a short time.

What is syphilis?

Once the syphilitic bacterium – treponema pallidum – has entered the body, it creates lesions, known as chancres (pronounced cankers). The first symptom, known as the primary symptom, will be a definite hard ulcer (chancre) at the site of infection, which usually appears two to three weeks after transmission. Secondary symptoms appear about two months after that and include:

- Fever.
- Tiredness.
- Lymph node enlargement.
- Faint red rash on the chest area.

After a lot longer, sometimes even years after initial infection, the syphilis enters what is called a tertiary (third) phase, which produces masses, similar to tumours, throughout.

'Syphilis is very similar and sometimes indistinguishable from other sexually transmitted infections.'

How do people catch syphilis?

Syphilis is transmitted through sexual intercourse with an infected person who has a syphilitic sore. These sores can be found mainly on or around the external genitalia of men and women, or in and around the anus. The sores can also occur around the lips and mouth, so transmission can occur through vaginal, oral or anal sex.

Myth busting facts!

You cannot contract syphilis from:

'Syphilis is passed from one person to another by direct contact with a chancre.'

- Toilet seats.
- Swimming pools.
- Shared clothing.
- Handles or doorknobs.
- Baths.
- Jacuzzis.
- Eating utensils.
- Shared food.

What symptoms should I be looking out for?

Unfortunately, a lot of people who are infected with syphilis sometimes do not have any symptoms for years. However, this does not mean that they are not at risk of later complications.

Transmission of syphilis will occur if you have sexual contact with anyone who has sores in the primary or secondary stages, yet because the initial sores are usually painless, they are often disregarded as being something else.

The primary stage

This first stage is often marked by the appearance of a single, often painless, sore (there may be more than one in some cases). Usually, this sore appears on average three weeks after the transmission of the bacteria, but it can be as early as 10 days or as late as three months. The chancre will look small and round, will often feel painless, yet firm to the touch, lasting three to six weeks and disappearing without any treatment. (Your lymph nodes may also enlarge around the site of the chancre.)

However, if treatment is not received for the syphilis bacteria, the infection can progress, creating further problems.

The secondary stage

Two months after the first infection, secondary symptoms begin to be noticed by the infected person. These symptoms include:

- A raised temperature.
- Tiredness and lethargy.
- General enlargement of lymph nodes.
- Red rash on the chest that lasts for about a fortnight.
- Sore throat.
- Some hair loss.
- Headache.
- Weight loss.
- Muscle pain.

The rash that appears can also be on other parts of the body, appearing as a red-brown rash that feels slightly rough, on the palms of your hands and the soles of your feet. This rash must always be checked out because you can also get a condition with this rash called pompholyx. This particular rash is not dangerous to your health, but can also be a chronic condition. Sometimes, however, the rash that comes with the syphilis is so faint, it is not noticed.

'Chancres are most often small and painless, lasting nearly two months and disappearing without treatment. However, the infection is still active in the body causing secondary damage.'

The symptoms of secondary stage syphilis will resolve themselves with or without treatment, but if you don't receive treatment, then the syphilis can and will progress to the tertiary stage.

The tertiary (third) stage

This last stage is often called the 'hidden' stage as it begins when the primary and secondary symptoms are disappearing. People without the knowledge contained in this book, may believe themselves to be cured and may feel relieved not to have to visit their doctor.

However, without treatment the infected person will continue to have syphilis in their body, even without signs or symptoms, and this stage can appear to last for years.

The late stages of syphilis develop in about 15% of the people who are not treated for it and usually begin one or two decades after the symptoms first appeared. The late stages of syphilis can cause masses (gummas – most commonly found in the connective tissue, testes, heart, bone and brain) in the body, disrupting and damaging the internal organs such as the:

- Blood vessels.
- Bones.
- Brain.
- Eyes.
- Heart.
- Joints.
- Liver.
- Nerves.

The signs and symptoms of late stage, untreated, syphilis infection are:

- Dementia.
- Difficulty coordinating muscles.
- Gradual blindness.

- Numbness.
- Paralysis.
- Death.

Tertiary syphilis as you can see may cause serious damage, even death, if left untreated. The damage to the heart and blood vessels is known as cardiovascular syphilis, but if it affects the brain or spinal cord, it is known as neurosyphilis. Neurosyphilis results in sufferers developing tabes dorsalis, which is where the infecting bacteria destroy the sensory nerves. Sufferers experience severe stabbing pains in their legs and body, have trouble staying upright and lose bladder control. Other symptoms of neurosyphilis are blindness, and general paralysis of the insane (deafness, epilepsy and dysarthria (speech disorder) may occur).

I'm pregnant. How will having syphilis affect my baby?

Syphilis infection and pregnancy do not mix well. The bacterium that causes the syphilis can infect the baby during the pregnancy and if you have been infected with syphilis for a long time during the pregnancy, then your baby is at risk of being stillborn or dying shortly after birth. The longer you have been infected, the higher the risk.

An infected baby may be born without signs or symptoms of the syphilis infection, but if the baby is not treated then it can run the risk of developing incredibly severe symptoms within a few weeks and again, if untreated, the baby may become developmentally delayed, experience seizures or even die.

How will a doctor test me for syphilis?

Sometimes syphilis can be easily diagnosed by examining a chancre with a special microscope called a 'dark-field' microscope, which specifically picks up the infectious syphilitic bacteria in the sore.

Another way to test for syphilis is through a blood test at a laboratory. After infection has begun, the body automatically produces antibodies to fight off the invasion of syphilis and the blood test picks up on these antibodies. A very low level of syphilis antibodies will stay in the affected person's blood stream for many months or even years after the disease has been treated with medication.

How will I be treated for syphilis?

There are many ways to treat syphilis and, in the early stages of the infection, it is relatively simple to cure.

If you have had syphilis for less than a year, you can be cured with a simple intramuscular (into the muscle) injection of penicillin (a drug used to treat bacterial infections.) There are few side effects, but some people may be allergic to penicillin and so it is important to notify your doctor if this is the case for you. If you do not know if you are allergic, signs and symptoms to look out for are skin rash, fever and swollen throat. If you are allergic, then there are other drugs that can be used to treat your syphilis infection.

If you have had syphilis for longer than a year, then you may need extra doses of penicillin. There is nothing you can take as a home remedy or over-the-counter medication that will cure your syphilis!

Any treatment you do take will kill the bacteria that cause the syphilis and prevent the infection from causing you any more harm, but it will not repair any of the damage already caused by the bacteria.

Other treatments for syphilis include:

* Doxycycline (trade name – Vibramycin, an oral medication).

* Erythromycin (trade name – Erymax or Erythrocin which can be administered orally, by injection or topically. Side effects are not common).

* Tetracycline (trade name – Achromycin. Side effects are common).

So once I'm treated, will I be cured forever?

Unfortunately not; just because you've treated your syphilis, it does not mean you are protected from ever getting it again. You can still be at risk, even with your antibodies.

How do I stop myself getting syphilis in the first place?

By abstaining from sex or being in a long-term monogamous relationship with someone whom you know is free of infection.

Abusing alcohol, binge drinking or using drugs can make you take risks sexually. Risks you wouldn't normally take if sober, like having sex with a stranger without using a condom.

When meeting someone new, who you are sure you are going to have sex with, make sure you ask them about their health history, what their HIV status is and whether they have ever been to a GU clinic and what for. If in doubt, or you do not trust what someone is saying, then do not have sex with them until you see a negative test result with their name on it from a registered clinic.

Remember that STIs such as syphilis and others (warts, herpes) can still be contracted by sexual partners, even if condoms are used. The disease can be active on the surface of the skin that is not covered by the condom and therefore transmission of disease still occurs. Condoms can reduce the risk, but not eliminate it.

If your partner tells you it is okay to have sex with them because they have washed themselves around their genitals or have douched recently, then they are wrong. That will not prevent the transmission of syphilis or any other STI.

If your partner has some obvious symptoms in the groin or rectal area, then do not have sex with them.

'Lots of people infected with syphilis do not have any symptoms for years, yet remain at risk from complications.'

Talking to a teenager about syphilis

Many teenagers may roll their eyes when you raise the subject of syphilis as many people today – and not just teenagers – believe that syphilis is something that happened in the world years ago, during the nineteenth century. Yes, it did happen then, but it is experiencing resurgence again today.

Syphilis does not just occur between homosexuals, but heterosexuals, too. It is important that your teenager knows the risks. Ensure they understand that using a condom will not protect them from syphilis. If they're going to have sex and spot anything unusual in a partner 'down below', then they must not have sex with that person, vaginally, anally or orally.

Syphilis infects the young as well as the old. They are not invincible. They are vulnerable if they take a risk. Tell them not to drink. Not to take drugs. Tell them they need to be sensible. Ask them if they have any questions and always make any sexual talk with your teenager a two-way street. You must be prepared to listen to them as much as you expect them to listen to you. Only then can you experience a true, honest communication, if you both show respect and do not shy away from telling the real truths because that is what teenagers want to hear.

■ No flowery language.

■ Be upfront.

■ Be honest.

■ And listen.

Factfile

In 2002, Portsmouth reported only nine cases of syphilis. Just four years later, this had rocketed by a massive 3,577% to 331 cases; an incredible difference. (*Portsmouth News*, 2007)

Nationwide, according to a report by the Health Protection Agency, there were 162 reported cases of syphilis (primary and secondary infections) in 1997. By the year 2000, this had doubled to 342 reported cases and by 2006, had increased yet again to a shocking 2766 cases of syphilis; an increase of 1,607%.

The HPA reported that in 2006, 51% of these diagnosed cases occurred between men who were having sex with other men, but the most recent increases have been between women and heterosexual men.

Bejel (endemic syphilis)

It is worth mentioning bejel here, even though it is not a typical UK syphilitic infection.

Bejel is usually reported in eastern Mediterranean countries and Northern Africa, but it is worth knowing about in case you have cause to visit these countries, or know someone from there.

Bejel is prevalent in areas where personal hygiene and availability of clean sanitation is low. The disease is most commonly reported among children and adults and is contracted through skin-to-skin contact. The first lesions appear in the moister areas of the body such as the armpits, groin and mouth. However, as the infection grows and takes a stronger hold of the body, the skin can be overtaken by wart-like bumps, especially in the anal and genital area.

Bejel is rarely fatal and is usually treated by penicillin.

Summing Up

- Syphilis can often be mistaken for other diseases so it is essential to get it properly diagnosed.

- The incidence rate of syphilis is massively increasing in our society today.

- Condoms will not protect you fully from syphilis.

- Syphilitic sores are called chancres.

- Pregnant women can put their unborn babies at risk if they have syphilis.

- There are three stages; primary, secondary and tertiary.

- Syphilis can be cured in the early stages but you can still be open to re-infection.

Chapter Six

Hepatitis A, B and C

Hepatitis (hep – a – tie – tiss) A, B and C are often abbreviated to HAV, HBV and HCV, meaning hepatitis A virus, hepatitis B virus and hepatitis C virus. All are contactable through sexual activity and each has different risks and symptoms.

What is hepatitis A?

HAV is the most common of the known viral hepatitis infections. Also known as epidemic hepatitis it is most frequently found in areas of low sanitation and hygiene. People drink or eat contaminated water or food and then the disease can be passed on sexually as the infection is found in the faeces of an infected person and those that participate in anal sex are then particularly at risk.

HAV affects both men and women of all age groups and, once exposed, symptoms can develop in as little as two weeks.

'Hepatitis A can occur where sanitation and hygiene are poor.'

What symptoms should I be looking out for?

Again, as with so many other infectious sexually transmitted diseases, infected people can show little or even no signs of infection, yet still be infectious to other people with whom they have sex. But of those that do have symptoms, the events to look out for are:

- Abdominal pain.
- Itchy skin.
- Jaundice (a yellowing of the skin or the whites of the eyes, which is a sign of excess bilirubin in the blood).
- Loss of appetite.

- Some flu-like symptoms.
- Sickness and diarrhoea.
- Weight loss.

So what will happen if I don't get this treated?

HAV infection usually clears up after a few months, though the infection may reoccur or persist for a long time in some people. Rarely, the symptoms can be so harsh that a sufferer requires monitoring in hospital. Permanent damage to the liver is also extremely rare.

How will a doctor test me for hepatitis A?

HAV is tested for by a blood test at your doctor's surgery or local GU clinic.

If my result is positive, what treatment will I have?

If your result is positive, then this means that you are either currently infected with HAV, or you have had a past infection. The antibody detected in the test will tell the doctor whether your HAV infection is active now.

If you test positive, you will be asked about your sexual history, who you have recently had contact with and which sexual partners may need to be tested too.

If your result shows that you have the antibodies to a past infection that has now cleared, then it will show that you are naturally immune to the HAV infection.

However, if your result is negative, a doctor may still suggest that you get yourself immunised, especially if you are in a high risk group.

Most people fight off the HAV infection naturally by themselves and find that they feel fully fit once again after a few months. Because of the natural effect the HAV has on your liver in particular, you may be advised to avoid certain foods and drinks in your diet, which will prevent your liver becoming inflamed. Rest is recommended, as is a healthy diet. Good hygiene should always be of paramount importance, so ensure that you wash your hands regularly, especially before eating and after using the toilet.

There are immunisations that can be given to patients with HAV or those who may be at high risk of contracting HAV. These immunisations take the form of a series of injections of gammaglobulin. Gammaglobulins are usually immunoglobulins, a type of protein found naturally in the blood, and an injection of this will provide temporary protection against HAV. A series of injections provides longer protection.

One injection in the arm gives protection for about a year and a second injection lengthens this protection for about a decade.

What is hepatitis B?

HBV is extremely similar to HAV symptom-wise, but is more problematic in that it can be a chronic (long term) illness, rather than a short term one.

How am I going to catch it?

Unfortunately, HBV is considered more infectious than human immunodeficiency virus (HIV). It is a very common infection and it is suspected that there are hundreds of millions of people infected worldwide.

HBV is most frequently passed on through the exchange of bodily fluids, therefore making sexual intercourse an ideal situation for the condition to be spread. However, sexual intercourse, whether vaginal, anal or oral, is not the only way it can be caught. You can also catch it through:

- Sharing needles.
- Using unsterilised equipment for body art or tattoos.
- An infected mother, passing it to her baby during the birth process.
- Being exposed to unclean blood.

It cannot be caught from:

- Being near someone who is sneezing.
- Being near someone who is coughing.
- Hugging.
- Faeces.

'Hepatitis B is a severe viral form of hepatitis transmitted in infected blood, causing fever and jaundice.'

So what are the symptoms of hepatitis B?

The mild symptoms are very similar to HAV. They include:

- Itchy patches of skin.
- Jaundice (yellow skin and whites of eyes, due to excess of bilirubin).
- Lack of appetite.
- Short flu-like symptoms.
- Sickness and diarrhoea.
- Weight loss.

'Hepatitis B is transmitted through infected blood or blood products such as those shared by drug users, or through sexual contact.'

If your symptoms become severe, then you will most probably be admitted to hospital for treatment and supervision.

So what will happen if I don't get treated?

If you have HBV for a long time, then you can develop chronic liver damage such as cirrhosis (which is a condition that cannot be cured) and liver cancer. There is a mortality rate of between 5-20%.

I'm pregnant. How does having hepatitis B affect me?

If you have HBV, then you can pass the infection on to your baby during the delivery process. If this is suspected, a baby can be immunised at birth to prevent the infection. However, if you do not realise you are infected with HBV, then your baby is at risk.

Newborn babies infected with HBV are more likely to become chronic carriers of the infection.

Need2Know

How will I be tested for hepatitis B?

A blood test at your doctors or GU clinic will confirm or deny your suspicions.

My result is positive. What does this mean for me?

Like HAV, a positive result may indicate a present or past infection. If it is a past infection, then this means that you have been infected with HBV, but your own body has successfully fought off the infection and you will have a natural immunity.

Your positive result may indicate that you are a carrier of HBV and that you are able to infect others, even if you have not shown any of the symptoms. Do not be complacent about this, however, as even without the mild symptoms, you are still at risk of developing the chronic conditions mentioned above.

My result is negative. What does this mean for me?

This means that you have never come into contact with the HBV infection and are not immune to it. If you suspect that you may have been exposed or that you are in a high risk group, then you may be advised to have a HBV immunisation.

So what treatment will I have?

If you have a positive test result, then you may receive further tests. These are usually carried out by a specialist doctor who is able to determine whether the HBV has badly affected your liver and what your best treatment would be. A small minority may need a liver biopsy (a biopsy is the removal of a small piece of living tissue).

Thankfully, the majority of HBV infected people will not have severe symptoms and a specific treatment may not be required, but this can only be confirmed after you have seen a specialist. You may be monitored by your doctor as your own immune system comes into play to fight off the infection in your body.

'Infectious hepatitis is caused by viruses and can be detected through blood tests.'

A few people will develop chronic HBV infection, mostly infants and newborns and these will receive anti-viral medication to help prevent damage to the liver. This medication may take the form of tablets or injections. Drugs used are usually Baraclude, Interferon Alpha (from white blood cells) and Lamivudine (also used to treat HIV infection).

Treatment lasts for about half a year and the patient will be advised to rest as much as possible, eat and live healthily and avoid alcohol.

Anyone who receives a positive test result should be advised to have regular blood tests to check on the virus and not to share anything that might transmit the virus. A condom must always be used during sexual intercourse.

What is hepatitis C?

This is a disease of the liver, transmitted through blood and blood products, e.g. sharing needles, or is passed from an infected mother to her baby during birth. If anyone has any fresh cuts or wounds to their genitals it can also be transmitted during sexual intercourse.

How am I going to catch it?

Usual transmission of HCV is through the transmission of blood or sexual intercourse and is said to be more prevalent than HAV or HBV. Drug users are at high risk, as are those who have unprotected sex.

It cannot be caught through casual contact such as hugging or being near someone with a cold.

So what symptoms should I be aware of?

Symptoms will not be immediately apparent when you become infected with HCV. Usually, you may not be aware that you have been infected until much later, say four or five months after infection. Look out for the following symptoms:

- Itchy patches of skin.
- Jaundice (yellowing of the skin or whites of the eyes due to excess of bilirubin).

- Lack of appetite.
- Short flu-like symptoms.
- Sickness and diarrhoea.
- Weight loss.
- Fatigue.
- Sore bones and joints.
- Dry eyes.

As you can see, many of the symptoms are the same as those for HAV and HBV.

What will happen if I don't get treatment?

One fifth of all HCV infected people will naturally fight the infection themselves but will not become immune. You can still be re-infected. The other four fifths will develop chronic (long term) HCV. The virus will stay alive and active in their bodies throughout their lives and they will always be infectious to others.

Complications include:

- Cirrhosis.
- Liver cancer.

How will a doctor test me for hepatitis C?

Tests for HCV have only been available for about twenty years now and are performed through a blood screening to detect antibodies.

My result is positive. What does this mean for me?

If you have a positive result then this means that the antibodies against HCV have been found in your bloodstream. You have been exposed to the virus and your immune system has reacted against it. It may also mean that you are a 'carrier' of HCV.

'Chronic hepatitis continues for months or years, eventually leading to cirrhosis of the liver.' Oxford Concise Medical Dictionary, 6th edition, OU Press.

After your first positive test, a specialist doctor will then test further by looking for the specific genetic markers of the hepatitis C virus to determine whether the virus is current or past. However, if it appears to be a past infection, then that does not mean that you are now immune.

My result is negative. What does this mean for me?

This means that you have never had HCV, nor have you been exposed to it. However, as it can sometimes take a while for the antibodies to appear and if you're worried that you have been exposed or infected, a doctor may suggest a retest at a later date and advise you to ideally abstain from intercourse, but to definitely always use protection.

My result is positive. What will my treatment be?

HCV mainly affects the liver, so a positive test result will indicate that doctors will want to ascertain how damaged, if at all, your liver is. Specialists usually perform two tests:

- Liver biopsy.
- Liver function test (LFT).

A liver biopsy

A doctor will insert a small, hollow needle through the abdomen and into the liver where a small sample will be taken. This sample will be thoroughly examined under a microscope to determine whether the liver has got any inflammation, scarring or cirrhosis.

A liver function test

This test specifically measures how the liver is working and is performed through another blood test. The blood is examined to see which enzymes and proteins are present in the blood and what their volumes are, to assess how effectively the liver is functioning.

Treatment for HCV has much improved but after treatment only a third to one half of treated patients will be successful in ridding themselves of the infection.

The drugs used are Interferon, which is less effective when used on its own and is taken orally, and Ribavirin (trade names – Rebetol and Virazole). Ribavirin is taken by way of an inhaler or by mouth. If it is thought that you require this drug then you should declare whether you also have HIV or are possibly infected with HIV, as it does not work well with some HIV drugs.

Unfortunately, there are some unpleasant side effects to these medicines, including, but not limited to:

- Aches and pains.
- Bacterial pneumonia.
- Breathing problems.
- Depression.
- Flu-like symptoms.
- Headaches.
- Nausea.
- Skin rashes.
- Tiredness.

As a patient you will undergo regular check-ups while being treated and once finished, it is important to make clear that if the infection has been beaten, it does not mean you are immune from getting it again.

Once 'clear' you will or should have regular check-ups and blood tests to ascertain your health in this regard. Alcohol, once again, should be avoided, as should anything that might put an undue strain upon your liver.

How can I protect myself against hepatitis C?

By abstaining from sex or by being in a long-term monogamous relationship with someone who is clear of the infection.

I've had it once, how do I stop it from happening again?

There is no true vaccine to this infection and, like other diseases, it can mutate and change its genetic make-up quickly and easily, making the discovery of a vaccine difficult. Therefore, the most you can do is to take all measures to prevent yourself from getting this again.

- Only have sex with a partner who you know is clear of infection.
- If you use drugs, then do not share needles or any other drug paraphernalia.
- Always use protection during sex.
- Don't share toiletries / shaving equipment or anything that may be tainted with blood.
- Ask your doctor what measures you ought to take.

Talking to a teenager about hepatitis A, B and C

It is important that teenagers know that these infections are on the rise and that anyone infected with the conditions, may not have obvious, apparent symptoms.

If they are going to have sex, then they must always make absolutely sure about the health and sexual history of their partner and should always use a condom.

It's an unfortunate fact that a lot of teenagers may have tried drugs and even if you have never raised this subject with your teen, then it is important to do so now. HAV, HBV and HCV can so easily be passed on in these ways, through sharing drug making equipment, needles, spoons, etc. Any item that could have some infected blood on or in it will provide a possible huge risk of infection against them.

Talk them through this chapter, or let them read it themselves and tell them to come to you afterwards if they have any questions, or so that you can talk it over. Make them understand that people can die from these infections. Dame

Anita Roddick died in 2007 from hepatitis C that she contracted through a blood transfusion she had in 1971. She was only 64 and still, otherwise, relatively fit.

Factfile

Cases of hepatitis C are definitely rising and in 2006 alone, rose by 10%. According to a report by the Health Protection Agency, there were 7,580 reported cases of HCV in England alone, which rose to 8,346 in 2006.

Summing Up

▪ Hepatitis infection can badly affect the liver.

▪ Hepatitis A is found in the faeces of someone infected with HAV.

▪ Symptoms can be mild or non-existent.

▪ Those infected should try to avoid alcohol or anything that puts undue stress on their liver.

▪ Hepatitis B is more likely to cause chronic (long-term) illness than hepatitis A.

▪ Hepatitis B is passed on through the exchange of bodily fluids.

▪ Hepatitis B is estimated to be more infectious than HIV.

▪ Hepatitis B can cause jaundice.

▪ Hepatitis C is mainly transferred through blood.

▪ Drug users are at high risk of HCV.

Chapter Seven

HIV and AIDS

Basically, HIV is a retrovirus that is ultimately responsible for AIDS. There are two types of HIV; HIV-1 and HIV-2. The second one is most commonly found in Africa.

What causes it?

HIV was first discovered in the early 1980s and was initially believed to be a disease confined to drug users and homosexuals; however, anyone can now be at risk if they have sexual contact with another person whose history they do not know.

The HIV virus essentially locates and destroys a group of lymphocytes (a type of white blood cell) in the body which are known as 'helper' T-cells (CD4 lymphocytes). When these T-cells have been destroyed, the body's immune system is weakened. If a chronic stage of infection by HIV is reached, then AIDS (acquired immune deficiency syndrome) sets in and allows the body to be open to all manner of infections and viruses, especially pneumonia.

'AIDS was first identified in Los Angeles in 1981.' Oxford Medical Dictionary, 6th edition, OU Press.

How am I going to catch it?

HIV is primarily transmitted through sexual contact and can affect both heterosexual and homosexual men and women. Children can be born with the infection if contaminated during pregnancy or birth. It can also be contracted through sharing drug paraphernalia.

The infection outside of a human body is extremely weak and cannot survive, so you cannot catch it through sharing objects used by a HIV infected person or by touching that person in a non-sexual way.

What symptoms should I be looking out for?

Symptoms can be greatly delayed and are therefore not obviously apparent. You may not even have any symptoms, nor think to get checked unless it is suggested by a past partner who has tested positive for the infection.

There are no obvious marks / spots / warts about the genitalia, so you cannot assume that someone is clear of the infection if they have none of these. A generalised illness or varying intensity can present itself first, usually affecting the lymph nodes in some way, so any signs such as swelling of the lymph nodes should be taken seriously and investigated.

'HIV is not a strong virus outside of the human body.'

Some people may experience generalised tiredness or diarrhoea. They may lose weight and find it difficult to concentrate. If AIDS itself takes hold, there may be lots of 'simple' infections such as colds, chest infections, etc, or even small tumours appearing on the body and face. This latter condition is known as Kaposi's sarcoma and they are malignant tumours that form in the skin's blood vessels and mark the epidermis with dark brown / purple blemishes or nodules. They grow slowly and can be treated with radiotherapy.

What will happen if I don't get treated?

If you suspect or even know that you have been infected with HIV and do not do anything about it, then you are putting yourself at high risk of AIDS and eventual death. This disease is fatal and your illness may be short or lengthy.

I'm pregnant. How does having HIV affect me?

HIV can be passed on from an infected mother to her child in utero, or during the birth process. It can be found in blood, cervical secretions, urine and breast milk. Consequently, it may be safer to deliver your child through a caesarean section and bottle feed instead of breastfeeding.

How will I be tested for HIV?

Through a simple blood test.

If my result is positive, what treatment will I have?

There are many antiviral drugs that may be prescribed for you and these can be used either singly, or, more commonly, in combinations until the right 'cocktail' has been discovered for you.

You may also be asked if you require counselling and this suggestion should not just be dismissed out of hand, but considered strongly as this disease can have a profound effect on the way people think about their lives and futures.

The drugs available are a combination of reverse transcriptase inhibitors and protease inhibitors.

Reverse transcriptase inhibitors

Reverse transcriptase is an enzyme (a protein) that is usually found in retroviruses, such as HIV. The inhibitors prevent the retrovirus from implanting its RNA (ribonucleic acid) into a cell's DNA. These include Zidovudine (trade name – Retrovir. It can be administered by mouth or by intravenous drip. There are unfortunately common side effects such as sickness, headache and insomnia), Didanosine (trade name – Videx. It can be taken orally, but may cause sickness and diarrhoea, headache and possible damage to the nerves) and Lamivudine (trade names – Epivir and Zeffix).

Protease inhibitors

Protease is an enzyme produced by the HIV virus that it uses to grow quickly in the body. The inhibitors most commonly used are Indinavir (trade name – Crixivan), Lopinavir (trade name – Kaletra), Nelfinavir (trade name – Viracept), Ritonavir (trade name – Norvir) and Saquinavir (trade names – Fortovase and Invirase).

These are all given orally and most common side effects include sickness and diarrhoea.

'AIDS related deaths have fallen dramatically since 1995 due to better drug combinations.' www.patient.co.uk.

How can I protect myself against it?

HIV is present in blood, blood products and body fluids such as semen from HIV positive people, so you must ensure that if you have sexual contact with a new partner you always insist on using a condom. Also, if you are a drug user, never share needles or drug paraphernalia with someone else. Free needles and condoms are available at some clinics.

'Health workers have to maintain a high standard of clinical practice to avoid inadvertent infection through needlestick injuries, blood or blood products.' Oxford Medical Dictionary, 6th edition, OU Press.

Talking to a teenager about HIV and AIDS

A lot of teenagers will think that HIV and AIDS are the same name for the same disease, so it is important that they know that the HIV is the infection you get which can eventually (but not always) become AIDS.

The conditions were highly publicised during the 1980s and 1990s and a lot of misconceptions were believed. It is essential that when talking with your teenager, you explain how the disease is transmitted and that they are not going to catch it by shaking an infected person's hand or by using their loo. The HIV virus does not survive well outside of the body so it is not sitting on a toilet seat or a door handle. It is not on an infected person's clothes. These misconceptions were actually believed during the hysteria when the disease first became 'known' and so it is essential that teenagers in particular, get an accurate message about this disease today. Insist that they use condoms if they are going to have sex.

Factfile

According to a report by the World Health Organisation (WHO), there have been over 60,000 reported cases of HIV infection in the UK since 1982, yet the number of AIDS-related deaths in the UK has fallen dramatically since 1995, due to improved treatment and medications to control 'viral loads'. (As stated on the website www.patient.co.uk/showdoc/27000684.)

You can get more information specifically about HIV and AIDS, the research, the medications and what is being done to help the lives of those affected by these conditions at www.bhiva.org (The British HIV Association) and at www.nat.org.uk (The National AIDS Trust).

The National AIDS Trust has created a 'HIV in Schools' pack in response to the need for information amongst young people. If you want to request one of these packs, or download it direct from the site, visit www.worldaidsday. org/help_schools.asp.

Summing Up

- There are two types of HIV; HIV-1 and HIV-2.

- HIV-2 is most commonly located in Africa.

- HIV and AIDS is not an infection confined to homosexuals and drug users.

- HIV is transmitted through sexual intercourse, shared drug paraphernalia and in some cases, in utero.

- Signs of HIV may not develop for some years.

- AIDS is ultimately fatal.

Chapter Eight

Other Infections

I have included this chapter to show that there are some other less well-known infections, though not all of them are only transmitted through sexual intercourse. A number of them can be caught through close skin-to-skin contact, but as sexual intercourse requires that, I thought they deserved a place here.

They are:

- Bacterial vaginosis (BV).
- Crabs/pubic lice.
- Scabies.
- Thrush.
- Trichomoniasis.

Crabs/pubic lice

A 'crab' is a parasitic louse of the genus phthirus pubis. It lives permanently in the pubic hair and causes a lot of irritation and embarrassment. It is quite a common parasite and has also been known to inhabit the eyelashes and armpit hair.

The lice themselves do not transmit any infection or disease, but their bites do cause a problem and irritate the host. Being infected by these lice is often called pediculosis and any constant scratching of the skin can cause secondary bacterial infections to gain entry to the skin and body, so scratching should be avoided as much as possible.

'A "crab" is a parasitic louse of the genus phthirus pubis. It lives permanently in the pubic hair and causes a lot of irritation and embarrassment.'

These lice are more often than not transmitted through the act of sexual intercourse, but can also be transmitted through stray hairs left on clothing, towels or lavatory seats.

Thankfully, getting rid of pubic lice is as easy as getting rid of head lice and many treatments are available from your local pharmacy. However, if you do get an infection from constantly scratching the bites, then do see your doctor.

Scabies

This is a highly contagious skin disease, caused by the itch-mite. Symptoms of infection are intense irritation of the skin with red papules (small, fleshy pimples).

The itch mite sarcoptes scabiei seems to make most infected people itch at night times, but there can also be secondary bacterial infections. The female mite burrows tunnels in the skin so that she can lay her eggs and when these hatch, the baby mites pass onto new hosts through close skin-to-skin contact.

If your itching is incredibly intense, then you may be allergic to the mite itself; its ova and its faeces, all which stay within your skin, unless treated. Sites of infection most commonly noted are the penis, the nipples and the skin between the fingers and thumb.

Treatment is thankfully simple. Scabicide is applied, usually this is Permethrin (trade name – Lyclear) which is a synthetic insecticide that can treat head lice, pubic lice or scabies. Malathion (trade names – Derbac-M, Prioderm and Suleo-M) is another insecticide and is also used to treat head lice, pubic lice and scabies. However, this drug may cause some skin irritation or allergic reaction.

The insecticides are applied to all areas of the body from your neck downwards, and even if only one member of your household is infected, everyone needs to be treated. Clothing and bedding can be washed as normal.

Thrush

Also known as candidosis or candidiasis. This is a common yeast infection mostly associated with women, though men can also be infected and retransmit it back to their partner each time they have sex.

It presents itself as thrush in the vagina, but it can also be present in the mouth or even in skin folds where the surface of the skin may be moist and warm. On the skin surface, a thrush infection will look like a reddened area with a white patch. In the mouth, it may present itself as white patches on the inner cheeks and tongue. In the vagina, it can produce intense itching and often a discharge that is thick and white. Thrush can also develop in the body when a person is taking some broad spectrum antibiotics.

Treatment is simple and can be taken in a number of ways; topically, orally or intravaginally. The medication is available from your local pharmacy but always consult your doctor to confirm that your infection is definitely thrush. It can reoccur in the body many times.

'Thrush is a common yeast infection mostly associated with women, though men can also be infected and retransmit it back to their partner each time they have sex.'

Trichomoniasis

This is a parasitic infection, caused by the trichomonas vaginalis parasite in the urinary tract or vagina.

It causes an inflammation of the tissues in and around the genitals and also causes a smelly vaginal discharge (vaginitis). The infection can be transmitted to men through sexual intercourse and then they will also experience a penile discharge from their urethra.

Metronidazole (trade names – Flagyl and Metrozol) can be administered by mouth and is an excellent treatment, but may cause an upset stomach.

Bacterial vaginosis (BV)

This infection is common in women of childbearing age and occurs when the balance of bacteria in the vagina is upset by an overgrowth of another type of bacteria.

Signs of BV are:

- Discharge.
- Burning sensation.
- Itching.
- Pain.
- Unpleasant smell.

You have an increased risk of developing BV if you:

- Douche.
- Have sex with someone new.
- Have multiple sexual partners.
- Use a coil.

Scientists are a little unsure as to why having sex seems to upset this balance, but it is known that you cannot develop BV from swimming pools, beaches, toilet seats, towels or touching other objects. But, it is clear that women who are virgins and have never had any sexual activity are rarely affected, making sex a possible culprit.

There can be complications in having BV. It will increase your risk of infection to most STIs; if you are exposed to the HIV virus, for example. Developing BV while pregnant can create some problems during gestation. A woman is more likely to have a premature baby or have one with a low birth weight. The BV can also sometimes affect the fallopian tubes and womb, causing a complication such as pelvic inflammatory disease (PID).

BV can be confirmed through a physical examination and then a laboratory test after a swab is taken.

This imbalance of bacteria can correct itself after time, but it is best to seek treatment so as not to expose yourself to PID complications. A woman with BV is not likely to infect her male partner, but if she has a female partner then the risk of transmission is high. Treatment is with Metronidazole.

Statistics

STI statistics 1997 - 2006 (UK only)

Year	Syphilis (primary and secondary)	Gonorrhoea (uncomplicated)	Chlamydia (uncomplicated)	Herpes (first attack)	Genital Warts (first attack)	All new diagnoses
1997	162	13,063	42,668	16,615	68,883	231,185
1998	139	13,212	48,726	17,248	70,291	244,282
1999	223	16,470	56,991	17,509	71,748	261,406
2000	342	21,800	68,332	17,823	71,317	284,035
2001	753	23,705	76,515	18,944	73,458	303,169
2002	1,258	25,599	87,592	19,426	74,991	324,196
2003	1,652	24,965	96,151	19,231	76,598	346,126
2004	2,282	22,321	104,733	19,073	80,055	363,248
2005	2,804	19,248	109,418	19,830	81,201	368,341
2006	2,766	19,007	113,585	21,698	83,745	376,508
% change (2005-06)	-1%	-1%	4%	9%	3%	2%
% change (1997-06)	1,607%	46%	166%	31%	22%	63%

All new episodes seen at GUM clinics: 1997-2006. United Kingdom and country specific tables, Health Protection Agency, July 2007.

© Copyright Health Protection Agency.

Table reprinted with the kind permission of the Health Protection Agency. Visit www.hpa.org.uk for more information.

It could be quite easy to dismiss a dry table of numbers, but these figures in the table above represent people. People who have been to clinics and got themselves treated.

How many haven't?

How many are wandering around, sleeping with other people, totally unaware that they have an infection?

It's a scary thought.

Not such a dry table of numbers now.

Summing Up

- A 'crab' lives in the pubic hair and causes irritation and embarrassment.
- Scabies is a highly contagious skin disease, caused by the itch mite.
- Thrush is mostly associated with women, though men can also be infected.
- Trichomoniasi is a parasitic infection, which can affect both men and women.
- Bacterial vaginosis (BV) is common in women of childbearing age.

Chapter Nine

Alcohol Abuse and the Rise in STIs

It is thought that the rise in youngsters that binge drink or abuse alcohol on a regular basis, is having a direct effect on the numbers of reported cases of sexually transmitted infections.

There can be no doubt that STIs are on the increase and because binge drinking has become somewhat of a 'culture' amongst teenagers and young adults, there is the association – they get drunk, they do not take precautions, such as condoms, and many of them cannot even remember having sex.

According to a survey of over 500 patients at a sexual health clinic in Portsmouth, a large amount of them admitted that alcohol contributed to the reasons for them being in the clinic.

Published in the *International Journal of STD and Aids*, the research reveals that nearly 90% of the respondents (almost 450) admitted that they far exceeded the government's suggested drinking levels of six units for women and eight units for men. Shockingly, almost 80% of those in the survey (nearly 400) stated that because of their alcohol consumption, they'd had unprotected sex as a result. Worryingly, only 14% of men and 18% of the women said that they always used a condom with a new partner. That means that 86% of the men and 82% of the women didn't.

During the three months that this survey took place, nearly 100 women reported a pregnancy and just over half of those stated that the pregnancy was not wanted and a third of them had been drinking heavily before having unprotected sex.

'It is thought that the rise in youngsters that binge drink or abuse alcohol on a regular basis, is having a direct effect on the numbers of reported cases of sexually transmitted infections.'

As we enter the 24 hour drinking culture, staff in sexual health clinics can only assume that the problems of STIs and abusing alcohol will increase, resulting in more people reporting cases.

So what can be done about this? Should schools include in-depth information about the effects of alcohol alongside sexual education? Should clear links be made to them?

Certainly the importance of condom use cannot be denied, but then young people should also be made aware, as earlier chapters stated, that condoms will not give you 100% protection against STIs.

'There is a clear, scientific link between drinking too much alcohol and taking increased sexual risks.'
Linda Tucker,
Consultant Nurse in
Sexual Health and HIV,
'Binge drinking not a
tonic for sex health',
Portsmouth News,
2007.

Alcohol is a depressant and though it is illegal to sell it to a minor, teenagers can still get their hands on it quite easily. Large groups of youths can be intimidating in today's society and when a member of the public is approached by a large group and asked if they would go and buy them some alcohol, the fear factor often means that they do so, helping to fuel the binge-drinking often associated with young people.

The alcohol slows down responses in a person's body, both physically and mentally and makes them less alert. Therefore, when a youngster who has been heavily drinking is approached for sex, they are less likely to stop and think carefully about the implications of unsafe sex. The alcohol makes them feel more confident, less shy and more popular and they think it'll be fun, which is how the problem can start. For more information on teenage and underage drinking, and its effects on the body, see *Alcoholism – The Family Guide*.

Chapter Ten

What Happens at a Genitourinary (GU) Clinic?

Many people have a stereotyped image of a GU clinic. Some may imagine a cold, sterile place, where people hide their faces behind magazines as they quietly wait to be taken away and examined. Others imagine that they are peopled by prostitutes and those in the sex industry and it's a dirty place to be. Perhaps the seats aren't even safe to sit on? None of these things are true.

GU clinics are very professional establishments that cater for males and females of all ages and they don't just deal with sexually transmitted infections.

Most people are worried about attending a clinic, especially for the first time. They think they will be embarrassed, or feel shameful, but most report that actually the experience is fine and it is just like going to your own GP.

Below is some information reprinted with the kind permission of www. embarrassingproblems.com, which explains what it is like at a GU clinic, what happens there and what you can expect from your visit.

Why go to a genitourinary medicine clinic?

- Staff at genitourinary medicine clinics are specially trained and experienced in genital problems. They also have a reputation for being kind, sympathetic and non-judgmental.

- As well as doctors and nurses, genitourinary medicine clinics usually have special counsellors ('health advisors') who can help you with worries, and give you additional information you may need.

- Genitourinary medicine clinics have facilities for doing tests for all genital infections. For many tests, they will be able to give you the results straight away, and the appropriate treatment.

- You do not need a letter from your family doctor to attend a genitourinary medicine clinic – you simply phone the clinic and make an appointment.

- Genitourinary medicine clinics are very confidential. They will ask if they can send the result of your tests to your family doctor, but if you refuse, they will not do so.

'GU clinics are very professional establishments that cater for males and females of all ages and they don't just deal with sexually transmitted infections.'

What sort of problems can the clinic help with?

You can attend a genitourinary medicine clinic for tests if you think you might have a sexually transmitted infection, whether or not you have symptoms (such as a discharge). You can attend the clinic to be tested for HIV. The clinic could also help you if you think something is wrong with the shape or appearance of your genitals.

Finding a genitourinary medicine clinic and making an appointment

There are several ways of finding your nearest clinic.

- The telephone number is probably listed in the 'Business and Services' section of your phone book under 'Venereal Diseases' or 'Sexually Transmitted Diseases' or 'Sexual Health'.

- You could telephone your local hospital and ask for information about the nearest genitourinary medicine clinic.

- For people in the UK, look at the Playing Safely website, which has a section on 'Where to get help' that lists your nearest clinic.

When you have located the clinic, telephone to make an appointment. You do not need a doctor's letter. When you telephone, ask for clear directions to find the clinic – genitourinary medicine clinics are often tucked away and difficult to find!

Before attending the clinic

- Have a look at the website at www.wellsafe.org, which describes a visit to a typical clinic.

- Make sure you know where the clinic is, and leave plenty of time to get there.

- If it is your first appointment, allow at least an hour and a half.

- Women should work out the date of their last menstrual period and when they last had a smear test, and jot them down – you will probably be asked for this information.

- Especially for a first appointment, men should try not to pass urine for two hours beforehand. This is because samples may be taken for infection at the urethra ('pee hole'), and if you have passed urine recently, the evidence could be washed away so the test might be inaccurate. If you are in the waiting room and feel you must pass urine before seeing the doctor, tell a nurse so the urine sample can be taken.

- Switch off your mobile phone.

- Resolve to be completely honest. The questions you will be asked are simply to help make an accurate diagnosis. If you fib slightly, because of embarrassment, it will be less easy for the doctor to diagnose and treat your problem.

What happens at the clinic

If it is your first visit, you will see a doctor. The doctor will talk to you in private, and will ask you about your symptoms (if any), your recent sexual contacts and various medical questions. The doctor will then examine you, and then the doctor or nurse will take samples for testing. Before taking the samples, the doctor or nurse will talk to you about them, and make sure that you are happy for them to be taken.

- A urine sample is always needed.

- In men, samples are usually taken from the opening of the urethra, from the anus and from the throat.

■ In women, samples are usually taken from the vagina, the cervix (neck of the womb at the top of the vagina), throat and sometimes the anus. To take a sample from the cervix, a speculum is put into the vagina (like having a smear).

All these samples will be examined under the microscope in the clinic by an expert technician, who will look for signs of infection. The samples will then be sent to the laboratory for further, more complicated tests. In most cases, the doctor will be able to tell you what is wrong, and give you treatment there and then. The treatment is free.

Blood samples are usually taken, after discussion with you, to test for syphilis and/or hepatitis. If you wish, the clinic can also test you for HIV. You will also be given an opportunity to talk to the counsellor ('health advisor'), who will give you more information about your problem.

Worries about the clinic

It will be embarrassing. Genitourinary medicine clinics are not at all embarrassing. The staff deal with genital problems all the time – it is their job. To them, the genital area is just an ordinary part of the body.

The waiting room will be full of seedy people. The other people in the waiting room are just like you – ordinary people who are worried and trying to sort a problem out.

I do not want to talk about my sex life. They will think I have had too many partners. The staff are not at all judgmental about people's lifestyles. They are more interested in making a diagnosis of your problem, and giving you the right treatment.

The tests will be painful. For women, the tests are not painful (unless you count a blood test as painful). For men, taking the sample from the opening of the urethra ('peehole') is uncomfortable, but it takes only a moment.

They will do a HIV test and I'm not sure if I want one. You will probably be asked if you would like a HIV test, and it will be explained to you properly. If you are not sure, no one will try to persuade you – you can always go back and have it done another time.

They will send a letter to my family doctor telling him/her things about my sex life that I don't want him/her to know. The clinic will ask you if you want the results of tests to be sent to your family doctor. Often this is a sensible thing to agree to, but if you do not wish it, they will not do so. The letter will not go into detail about your sex life – it will probably be a short letter explaining the results. If you are worried, ask the doctor to tell you what information will be in the letter.

There will be medical students there. Clinics often do have medical students, because they have to learn about genital problems in order to become useful doctors. There will be one or two, not a huge group. They are bound by the same rules of confidentiality as everyone else in the clinic. The students are usually exceptionally sympathetic to people attending sexual health clinics, and may in fact make your visit nicer. However, if you would prefer not to have students there just say so.

For more information visit www.embarrassingproblems.com

Summing Up

A strange situation – like going to a GU clinic – can be frightening simply because it is something unknown and people can be all too taken in by horror stories and gossip, or possible imaginings of what these places are like. Hopefully, the myth-busting has helped clear your mind and made you feel more confident about approaching the clinic and the staff inside.

Just remember:

- No-one is judging you.

- They are there to help.

- Delays in your treatment can have serious complications for your future health and fertility in some cases.

Chapter Eleven

Meeting Someone New

Things I should remember

In today's society there are more and more ways to meet new people. Gone are the days where relationships began because people had met at bars and clubs.

Today there is speed-dating, the internet, email, MySpace, Facebook and others like them and it is all too easy to think that you know someone well.

'I met this guy through the internet. He sounded great. Really interesting and – what I thought was most important at the time – really good-looking. He'd sent me this pic of himself and he was well cute! Anyway, we "'talked" to each other for a few weeks and I thought I was falling for him. When he said he'd be coming to London with some mates and could we meet, I thought "great". He was exactly like his photo and I couldn't believe my luck. Within an hour of meeting we were walking around Covent Garden arm in arm and by evening I felt like I'd known him all my life. Big mistake. I didn't know him at all. Long story short, I ended up with a disease. I'd had sex with him at his mate's bed-sit. A really grotty place but because I thought this guy cared, I let him do it, believing it would lead somewhere. He disappeared real quick afterwards. I'd been nothing to him and it left me wondering how many other girls he'd done it to. At least my disease was treatable, but it could have been a lot worse.'
16 year-old girl.

The girl above made a few classic mistakes. She got taken in by the excitement of a possible relationship with a good-looking young man. She saw his good looks and read his funny, caring and considerate emails and thought that from those alone, she knew him well. So when they met 'in the flesh', so to speak, she'd already convinced herself that they'd known each other longer than they had. They were together one afternoon – a few hours – and by the evening were having sex which left her with chlamydia. She went to her doctor to get treated, but felt that she couldn't tell her parents. She was too ashamed to admit to them what she'd done. That she'd made a mistake. An error in judgement. What if they grounded her? Took away her computer? Withheld privileges? The idea of her father's anger and her mother's upset stopped her from letting them know how carelessly she put her life in danger.

Social networking sites and the internet have made it incredibly easy for people to get connected. We don't have to rely on telephones, physical meetings and handwritten letters anymore as the only way to stay in contact with each other. And they can also be great fun. But they can also create an easy to believe intimacy between people that isn't really there and so when e-buddies actually physically meet, it can be incredibly easy for them to think that they know the person they are with intimately.

But what have you asked them really?

Do you know their sexual history?

Just because someone tells you they've only slept with one other person, it doesn't mean that person is clean of disease. Just because someone tells you they've only been in one long-term relationship, it doesn't mean that they've never had a sexually transmitted infection.

It's all too easy to get excited at the start of what seems like a relationship and with teenage girls especially, the need to be liked can be quite strong and they can sometimes give in to pressures they wouldn't normally concede to. Teenage boys can also feel the need to brag about conquests if their mates are doing so and feel that they ought to sleep with as many people as possible.

This situation is not just confined to young people. Adults in middle and senior years are just as easily duped into sleeping with someone whose history they don't really know, but think it's okay because 'they seem so nice'. Well, nice people get STIs too.

So what can you do?

- Meet someone new in a public place.
- Always let someone else know where you'll be.
- Ask about past partners.
- Ask if they've ever been tested for STIs.
- Ask for their status and don't be afraid to do so. A moment of awkwardness is better than a lifetime's regret.
- Remember that STIs can be transmitted orally, vaginally and anally.
- Always use a condom.
- If in doubt, don't have sex.
- If you suspect an STI of your own, don't have sex. Have treatment.
- Don't be pressured into doing something you don't want to do.
- Don't drink to excess.
- Don't take recreational drugs.
- Be safe.

Chapter Twelve

Correct Condom Use

It may seem a simple matter of putting on a condom, and a lot of people assume they know what to do. But are you really sure you know what you're doing? Below are instructions for correctly using both male and female condoms.

The male condom

Male condoms are manufactured in a large variety of shapes and designs. There are two types of tips:

- A reservoir tip.
- A plain tip.

Reservoir tips allow for the ejaculate to be collected in one place after orgasm, whereas plain tip condoms are round-ended condoms, without a reservoir to collect.

You must use a condom every time you have sex and you must never use the same condom twice. Only put a condom on when the penis is fully erect to ensure a good fit and before the penis makes contact with the other person's genitals. (If you are having both anal as well as vaginal intercourse, a different condom must be used for each.)

How do I put the condom on?

- Check the expiry date to make sure the condom is fit for use.
- Open the condom packet carefully so as not to rip the condom inside.
- Place the condom on the head of the penis.

'You must use a condom every time you have sex and you must never use the same condom twice.'

- If it has a reservoir tip, hold the tip in one hand (this allows for the semen to be collected).

- Ensure the foreskin is back before rolling the condom down the length of the penis to the base.

- Make sure there are no trapped air bubbles.

- If you need lubrication, add it to the outside of the condom, using only water-based lubricants (KY Jelly, etc).

- When ejaculation has occurred, hold the condom as you withdraw from your partner so no semen can escape.

- Gently remove the condom and dispose of correctly by wrapping it in tissue and placing it in a bin and not flushing it down a toilet.

- If your condom breaks during intercourse, take it off and use another one.

- If the condom breaks and your partner is female, make sure she sees her doctor for emergency contraception.

What should I know about condoms?

- Different types are available – ribbed, flavoured, coloured, latex or polyurethane (for those allergic to latex).

- Latex condoms are generally considered more reliable.

- Use only with water-based lubricants, not oil-based as the oil breaks down the latex.

- Some lubricated condoms are lubricated with Nonoxynol 9 and some people can have an allergic reaction to this.

- There is no age limitation for purchasing condoms and family planning clinics as well as sexual health clinics will provide condoms for free.

- Approved condoms carry the British Standard Kite Mark or the EEC Standard Mark (the letters CE).

- Condoms have expiration dates so check your packet before use.

- Condoms can deteriorate if not stored properly.

- You can buy thicker condoms which are much stronger if you are having anal intercourse.

- Condoms are very effective at preventing HIV and other STIs, but are not 100% effective.

- Latex condoms are not biodegradable (but there are some manufacturers who produce biodegradable condoms, such as the UK company Zeneca Bio Products (formally ICI).

- Polyurethane condoms are not biodegradable.

- Condoms are most reliable as a method of birth control.

- If you have never used a condom before, practice putting them on and taking them off.

- Be proud to buy condoms. It shows that you are taking responsibility for your actions.

Excuses, Excuses...

Along the way, you might meet someone who could try to dissuade you from using a condom. If this happens, then always say no. If sex is going to happen, then a condom is going to get worn!

Some partners may act upset that perhaps you don't trust them, but trust can have nothing to do with it. In earlier chapters we came across many STIs where infected people don't realise that they have infections. What if this partner is one of those people?

A partner may say 'If you loved me, you wouldn't use a condom'. Love has nothing to do with it. You could love them to the ends of the earth, but are you going to risk your health, future and fertility because of it?

Using condoms may not appear to be sexy, but with a little practice, they can become a good part of love-making, especially if you get your partner to put the condom on you instead of doing it yourself. Knowing that you are both being as sensible as you can be, will make you both more relaxed which can only help matters!

Of course it can be very tempting in the heat of the moment to think 'oh, it won't hurt this once to do it without one', but is that momentary excitement worth risking everything for? And it could be 'everything', if you contract one of those life-threatening STIs.

Condoms will help prevent pregnancy, protect you both from disease, make little mess, are easily disposed of and have absolutely no side effects!

Don't be afraid to bring up the subject of condoms. They could save your life.

The female condom

The female condom is not so well known about and there is often a lot of misinformation about how they should be used. In fact a lot of young people may feel embarrassed at asking how to use them, so here is a little guide to help you on your way.

How do I use the female condom?

Original FC and FC2 sheaths

- Open the packet carefully, making sure you do not rip or tear into the packaging.
- Find a comfortable position for insertion.
- Make sure the inner ring is at the closed end of the sheath and then hold the sheath so that the open end is hanging down and away from you.
- Squeeze the inner ring and insert the sheath into your vagina, ensuring you can feel it goes up.
- Push the inner ring in as far as you can (it can help to insert a finger into the sheath to do this, being careful not to tear it).
- Make sure the sheath is not twisted, but lies straight.
- The outer ring should still be visible outside of the vagina.

VA female condom

- Hold the sponge and frame together and place the closed end into the vagina as far as you can.

- Check the sponge has opened up inside and is flat, rather than squashed.

- The frame should remain outside of the vagina.

- In both cases, the penis should be inserted into the sheath carefully for intercourse to take place.

- Do not use female condoms and male condoms together because the friction may cause a breakage.

- To remove the condom, twist the outer part gently and slowly pull out the sheath so no semen escapes.

- Wrap the sheath in tissue and dispose of in a bin, not down the toilet.

- Do not wash out and reuse female condoms.

Summing Up

- There are different types of condoms available.
- You must use a condom every time you have sex.
- Never use the same condom twice.
- Be proud to buy condoms.

Chapter Thirteen

Talking to Your Teenager

Slang

It can be intimidating to think you have to talk to your teenager about sex, especially if half the time, you don't know what they're talking about!

Some parents say their children seem to be talking another language; that they have these slang terms that seem to constantly change and they can't keep up with what they mean.

An extremely useful website for parents who wish to solve this problem is www.urbandictionary.com. It contains a useful alphabetical list that is constantly updated with current 'hip and happening' slang terms, used by teenagers in today's society.

Below is a tiny selection:

- I'm banging (I'm having sex with).
- I'm gonna bounce her (I'm not going to be her boyfriend anymore).
- Chicks (girls/women).
- Clowning around (a tease).
- He's got a full house (he's got both syphilis and gonorrhoea).
- We're gonna have some giblet pie (we're going to have sex).
- She's hot (I fancy her).
- We could hook up (we could get together).
- She's peeing glass (she's got an infection).
- He's trashed (he's drunk).

The thing to remember when talking with your teenager is not to use the slang terms yourself. You could end up using it wrong and looking idiotic and then your son or daughter is not very likely to want to take you seriously. They'll be too busy laughing at you!

Other ways to learn their 'language' is to keep up with what music they're listening to or what their favourite television programmes are. Become familiar with what your child surrounds themselves with and perhaps use music or TV as an opener to the conversation you want to have with them.

Help List

Avert

4 Brighton Road, Horsham, West Sussex, RH13 5BA
info@avert.org
www.avert.org
Avert is an international AIDS charity, but this wonderful site has plenty of information about all of the other STIs as well as statistics, history, quizzes, stories and a section for teenagers.

Centres for Disease Control and Prevention (CDC)

www.hivtest.org
A US website provided by CDC with information about HIV and AIDS testing, living with HIV and/or AIDS and a very good FAQ page. Visit www.cdc.gov for more information about CDC.

Condom Essential Wear

Helpline: 0800 567 123
www.condomessentialwear.co.uk
A website with information about sexual health and condom wear. Call the helpline for free confidential sexual health advice.

Cool Nurse

www.coolnurse.com
An American site, easily applicable to the UK, aimed directly at teenagers. Easily negotiable, it has a great, colourful layout, with no techno-babble, all about STIs. There are other links on the site that will help you learn about other health issues such as puberty worries, skin care, substance abuse, taking care of teeth, getting a good night's sleep, eye care and acne problems.

Embarrassingproblems.com

www.embarrassingproblems.com
This website is provided by Health Press Limited. It provides lots of 'straight talking' information on a range of personal health issues, including sexual health. Information is also provided on visiting the doctors and clinics.

The Family Planning Association (FPA)

UK office
50 Featherstone Street, London, EC1Y 8QU
Helpline 0845 122 8690 (9am to 6pm Monday to Friday)
Northern Ireland
Helpline 0845 122 8687 (9am to 5pm Monday to Thursday, 9am to 4.30pm Friday)
www.fpa.org.uk
The FPA helps people in the UK to make informed choices about sex. Their website is aimed at increasing education about sexual health. For free information and advice on sexual issues, including STIs call their helpline. The website also includes separate telephone numbers and addresses for Wales, Scotland and Northern Ireland.

The Herpes Virus Association

info@herpes.org.uk
www.herpes.org.uk
A website for the Herpes Virus Association. It has a very good FAQ page.

Kid's Health

www.kidshealth.org/parent/infections/std/talk_child_stds.html
This is a great site aimed at parents who want to know how to talk to their kids about sexual health and STIs; a great resource for those who believe in positive parenting.

www.likeitis.org.uk

This site is full of sexual health education aimed at young people and how they can protect themselves from STIs (which this site calls 'lovebugs'!). It also has a 'Dear Doctor...' page where common questions are asked and regularly updated.

NHS - Live Well

www.nhs.uk/livewell

A website where you can learn about sex, sexual health, STIs and much, much more. It has many links and it is a very easy to navigate site, giving information simple and clearly.

www.playingsafely.co.uk

Funded by the UK government Department of Health, this site has information about STIs, where clinics are local to you and the best way to get help for yourself.

R u thinking?

Tel: 0800 28 29 30

www.ruthinking.co.uk

A site about sexual facts, advice and answers. You can call the free helpline for confidential advice.

Sex, etc.

www.sexetc.org

A website with answers to sexual questions by teenagers and a range of other non-sexual health information too.

www.sexualhealth.org.uk

A great site covering general information on sexual health with a section for children still in school.

www.sexsense.co.uk

A website with some very sensible tips and advice about having sexual intercourse.

www.smartersex.org

This website is all about sexually transmitted infections and sexual health and it does a good job of clearing up many misconceptions about sex and STIs. There is also a page where you can test your own knowledge of sexual health, aimed at young people, so perhaps you could get your teenager to take the test and see what they know.

Terence Higgins Trust

Central office, 314-320 Gray's Inn Road, London, WC1X 8DP
Tel: 020 7812 1600
info@tht.org.uk
www.tht.org.uk
The website of the Terence Higgins Trust offers information, support and advice about living with HIV and AIDS. Click on the map for centres near you.

One last word

Not everyone will have had the chance to have entered a sexual relationship willingly and for those people who may have been raped or abused, there is a place where you can call if you need help and information.

The Rape Crisis Federation has a telephone number that is confidential. The calls are free and will not show up on your telephone bill. It is open Monday to Friday 9.30am – 4.30pm.

The Rape Crisis Helpline 0115 900 3560

Visit www.rapecrisis.org.uk for details of Rape Crisis groups near you.

ChildLine also has a helpline you can call that is free, confidential and will not show up on a telephone bill. Its website is full of information about anything that affects children and is well worth a look. Visit www.childline.org.uk.

ChildLine 0800 1111 (These calls are also free from a mobile phone.)

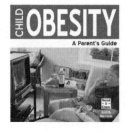
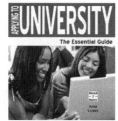
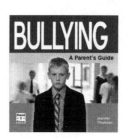
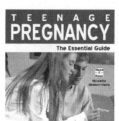
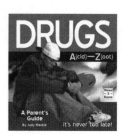